Ketogenic Diet

A 30-Day Quick-Start Guide To Losing Weight Fast

On A Low Carb, Ketogenic Diet

Maria Lively

Copyright Notice

No part of this report may be reproduced or transmitted in any form whatsoever, electronic, or mechanical, including photocopying, recording, or by any informational storage or retrieval system without expressed written, dated and signed permission from the author. All copyrights are reserved.

Disclaimer and/or Legal Notices

The information provided in this book is for educational purposes only. I am not a doctor and this is not meant to be taken as medical advice. The information provided in this book is based upon my experiences as well as my interpretations of the current research available.

The advice and tips given in this course are meant for healthy adults only. You should consult your physician to insure the tips given in this course are appropriate for your individual circumstances.

If you have any health issues or pre-existing conditions, please consult with your physician before implementing any of the information provided in this course.

This product is for informational purposes only and the author does not accept any responsibilities for any liabilities or damages, real or perceived, resulting from the use of this information.

Copyright © 2016 Maria Lively
All rights reserved.

CONTENTS

Part I: Understanding The Ketogenic Diet

1. What is the Ketogenic Diet? — 6
2. The History Behind the Ketogenic Diet — 8
3. The Top Benefits of Eating a Ketogenic Diet — 11
4. Understanding the Basics of Ketogenic Nutrition — 19
5. Mistakes to Avoid on a Ketogenic Diet — 23

Part II: Getting Started

6. Tips for Starting a Ketogenic Diet — 29
7. Grocery List for Foods You Should Be Eating — 31
8. 15 Super Convenient Breakfast Recipes — 33
9. Top 15 Lunch-On-The-Go Recipes — 34
10. Top 15 Delicious Dinner Recipes — 64
11. Convenient Keto Snacks — 87

Part III: Sticking With It

12. Goals & Mindset for Maintaining a Ketogenic Diet — 90
13. A System for Easily Preparing Your Meals For the Week — 92
14. How to Deal with Temptations and Sugar Cravings — 94
15. How to Handle Social Pressure — 99
16. Options for Eating Out at Restaurants — 103

Want 4 Free Reports That Will Make The Ketogenic Diet a Breeze?

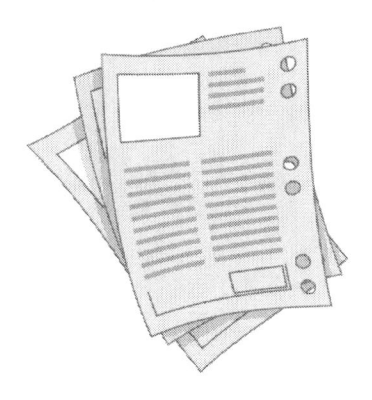

$17 Value!

The #1 reason people don't stick to a ketogenic diet is because they are tired of eating the same things over and over. That is why I have prepared 4 FREE PDF reports that will make sure you never get tired of sticking to the ketogenic diet.

I have taken the grocery list and recipes found in this book and have compiled them all into printable files that you can download, print, and take with you to the grocery store or kitchen to ensure that you always have variety and tasty foods in your diet.

Go to **http://bit.ly/1V24Kjf** to instantly download your $17 gift

Part One

Understanding the Ketogenic Diet

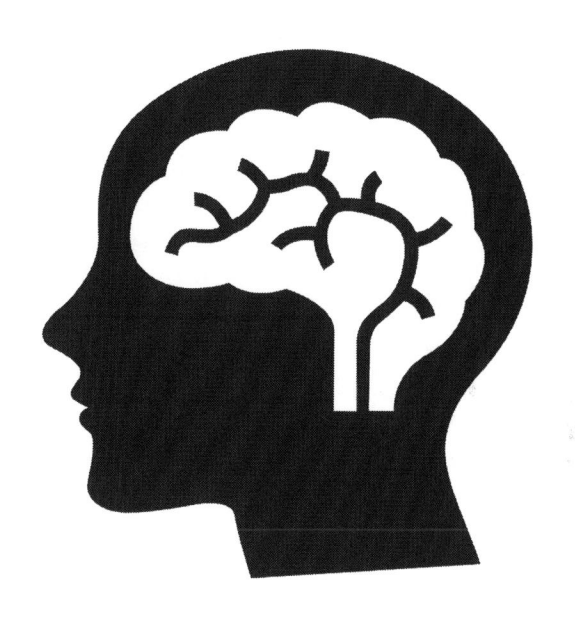

Chapter 1
What is the Ketogenic Diet?

The ketogenic diet is a specialized diet that was designed to help epileptic patients who were unresponsive to the routine medications given to them. Now the ketogenic diet is used by millions of people to lose weight and feel great. The typical ketogenic diet is as follows:

1) High in fat content

2) Adequate in protein

3) Low in carbohydrates

This particular diet is called the "ketogenic diet" because it actually makes the body think that the individual is fasting, which results in the body producing **ketones**. When the body is in what is deemed as "starvation mode," it begins to burn fats instead of carbohydrates. In the ketogenic diet, the primary energy source is fats. When this is combined with low amounts of carbohydrates being ingested, the body begins to produce more ketones and therefore, burns more fat.

In the typical diet, food gets converted into glucose, which then travels through the body and is used as energy. Typically, the brain uses glucose as a source of energy. However, when there are not enough carbohydrates available, the liver begins to process the fats to provide the brain with necessary energy in the form of ketone bodies and fatty acids. As the levels of ketone bodies begin to increase in the blood, the body enters **ketosis**. Several studies have revealed that when epileptic patients entered ketosis, they experienced a reduction of seizures when no other treatment seemed to be effective. Other individuals in ketosis are noted for experiencing clearer thinking, higher levels of energy, and increased happiness levels.

The ketogenic diet is comprised of just enough protein for body repair and growth. Additionally, the calories in the diet are enough to help an individual maintain a healthy weight for their age and height.

In the standard ketogenic diet, the ratio of proteins and carbohydrates to fats is 1:4. This means you should be eating 4x more fat as you are protein and carbohydrates. Sounds pretty good right? Some foods that are high in fat include cream, lard, duck fat, olive oil, and butter. Some of the foods containing high amounts of carbohydrates that should be avoided include sugar, bread, starchy fruits, grains, and pasta.
In the next chapter, we will discuss the history behind the ketogenic diet. Also, you will find in the first section of this book the top benefits of a ketogenic diet, understand the basics of the ketogenic diet, and some common mistakes to avoid when deciding to start a ketogenic diet.

Chapter 2
The History Behind the Ketogenic Diet

In the 1920s-1930s, the ketogenic diet became quite popular as treatment for patients with epilepsy. It was originally developed as an alternative to other therapies such as non-mainstream fasting. When anticonvulsant therapies were introduced, the ketogenic diet was left behind. However, even though the medications were quite effective for most patients, there were approximately 20-30 percent of epileptics remaining that were still experiencing the effects of epilepsy. Therefore, the ketogenic diet was reintroduced as a method for managing this condition.

The function of fasting in treating specific diseases has been known to mankind for thousands of years. The ancient Greek and ancient Indian physicians studied this therapy. "On the Sacred Disease," part of the early Hippocratic Corpus, described how making changes in diet could effectively manage the signs and symptoms of epilepsy. Additionally, the same author of this paper, also wrote "Epidemics," in which he described how a man abstained from consumption of drinks and food and was completely cured of all signs and symptoms of epilepsy.

The premier modern scientific study on fasting to cure epilepsy was done in 1911 in France. At this time, the primary treatment for epilepsy was potassium bromide. However, this treatment actually drastically slowed the mental capabilities of patients. As a result, twenty patients suffering from epilepsy were chosen and were put on a low-calorie, vegetarian food plan, in conjunction with fasting. While most of the patients were unable to adhere to this plan, two of the twenty patients did and showed some remarkable improvements. Additionally, when compared with the effects of the potassium bromide treatment, the changes in diet were shown to improve the mental capabilities of the patients.

So how does a ketogenic diet prevent seizures? In America during the 20th century, Bernarr Macfadden made the idea of fasting to restore health extremely popular. Hugh Conklin, a student osteopath of Macfadden's suggested fasting as a way to control the signs and symptoms of epilepsy. He proposed that the seizures related to epilepsy were due to a toxin that was being secreted in the intestine. He suggested that fasting for eighteen to twenty-five days could result in this toxin dissipating from the body, which would decrease, and potentially prevent, the seizures.

Conklin took a group of epileptic patients and put them on a "water diet." His findings were that 90 percent of children with the condition and 50 percent of adults were cured of their epilepsy. Later, an analysis of this study was performed, which showed that approximately 20 percent of the patients became seizure-free, and approximately 50 percent of those showed improvement.

In 1916, fasting as a mainstream treatment for the condition of epilepsy was adopted. According to the New York Medical Journal, Dr. McMurray reported that since 1912, he had been successful at treating his epileptic patients with fasting and a diet that was free of starch and sugar.

In 1921, endocrinologist, Rollin Woodyatt, took note that three water soluble compounds, acetoacetate, acetone, and hydroxybutyrate, collectively known as **ketone bodies**, were produced as a result of starvation or if the patient followed a diet low in carbohydrates and rich in fats. A physician named Russel Wilder, of the Mayo Clinic, referred to this as the ketogenic diet and began using it to treat epileptic patients.

In the 1960s, more research began to uncover the fact that ketones are produced per unit of energy by MCTs, or **medium-chain triglycerides**, due to the fact that they are quickly transported to the liver through the hepatic portal vein instead of going through the lymphatic system.

Then, in 1971, a ketogenic diet was devised by Peter Huttenlocher, where around 60 percent of the calories were from MCT oil. This allowed more carbohydrates and proteins to be included in the diet- which meant that parents were able to prepare much more enjoyable meals for their epileptic children. Many of the hospitals began to adopt this MCT diet instead of following the original diet - and some actually used a combination of the two.

Chapter 3
The Top Benefits of Eating a Ketogenic Diet

Over the decades, the ketogenic diet has stirred up extreme controversy. High-fat diets were often demonized by health professionals and the media who were afraid of fats- often referred to as "fat-phobic." Most people believed that the low-carbohydrate/high-fat diets would actually cause heart disease and elevated cholesterol levels in those who followed them.

However, now things are much different. Since 2002, more than 20 different studies on low-carbohydrate diets have been done on humans. In nearly every one of these studies, these low-carbohydrate diets come out way ahead of the diets they are being compared to. The truth is, not only do the low-carbohydrate diets result in much more weight loss, but they also lead to some significant improvements in most other health risk factors, including cholesterol, epilepsy, and more.

This chapter will provide the top 10 proven health benefits of following a low-carbohydrate, or ketogenic diet.

1) Ketogenic diets will actually kill your appetite - but in a good way.

The truth of dieting is that the single worst side effect is hunger. People always start a diet with the best of intentions, but then hunger gets the best of them. They begin to feel miserable and deprived, so they give up.
Studies have consistently proven that when individuals begin to cut carbohydrate levels in their diet and begin to add more fats and proteins, they actually consume fewer calories.

One gram of carbohydrate and protein contain 4 calories each. One gram of fat contains 9 calories. This means that fat is more calorically dense and therefore, more satiating. Also, have you ever eaten something sugary and instantly craved more of it? By consuming very little carbohydrates and sugar, these over-eating cravings begin to dissipate.

The bottom line is this: when people cut their carbohydrates, their appetite will reduce automatically and they will end up eating fewer calories without even noticing.

2) Ketogenic diets actually result in more weight loss than low-fat diets.

The truth is that one of the most effective, and simplest, ways to lose weight is to cut carbohydrate consumption without over-consuming fats and proteins. Many studies have proven that people who cut carbohydrate consumption actually lose more weight at a much faster rate than individuals who are on a low-fat diet. This is even true when those on the low-fat diets are actively restricting their caloric consumption.

One of the main reasons for this is that those on low-carbohydrate diets actually get rid of water weight due to the lowered insulin levels in their bodies. When insulin levels are lowered, the kidneys shed the extra sodium in the body, which can lead to drastic weight loss in the first couple of weeks.

When making a comparison of ketogenic diets versus low-fat diets, those on the ketogenic diets typically lose two to three times more weight without experiencing much hunger.

Though it is referred to as a diet, you should never think of a ketogenic diet as a "diet" but more so as a change in your lifestyle. The problem is, after about six months, "dieters" start giving up and will go back to eating the same junk. This causes their weight to start creeping back up. After all, the only way to successfully lose weight or to control a particular condition is to stick to it. However, if your goal is to lose a certain amount of weight, it is possible that you can start adding in healthy carbohydrates after you've reached your goal. In part 3 of this book we will discuss strategies you can use to stick to the ketogenic lifestyle, if you wish.

The bottom line is this: almost always, a ketogenic diet will lead to more significant weight loss than other diets, especially within the first six months.

3) In a ketogenic diet, most of the fat loss comes from the abdominal area.

Not all fat is created equally. There are good fats and there are bad fats. Also, where the fat is stored determines how it will affect our risk of diseases and our overall health.

In your body, you have subcutaneous fat, which is found under the skin and you have visceral fat, which is found in the abdominal area.

The visceral fat often lodges around organs and having a lot of this fat in your abdominal area can increase inflammation and insulin resistance. In addition, visceral fat is believed to be one of the main causes of metabolic dysfunction that is so common today.

Ketogenic diets are extremely effective for reducing this harmful fat. Not only do ketogenic diets result in more overall weight loss than their low-fat counterparts, but most of the fat that is lost comes from the abdominal cavity.

Over time, this can possibly result in a reduced risk of developing type 2 diabetes, heart disease, and other deadly diseases.

The bottom line is this: most of the fat lost on a ketogenic diet comes from the harmful visceral fat located in the abdominal area that has been proven to cause significant metabolic problems.

4) Ketogenic diets result in a reduction in triglycerides.

The medical community has proven that fasting triglycerides, the amount of fat molecules in the blood overnight, are a significant risk factor for heart disease. The main reason these triglycerides are elevated are from the consumption of carbohydrates, especially the simple sugar called fructose.

When people cut carbohydrate consumption by going on a ketogenic diet, they will typically see an extreme reduction in triglycerides in their blood.

The bottom line is this: a ketogenic diet is extremely effective for reducing blood triglycerides, which are fat molecules that have been proven to cause elevated risk factors for heart disease.

5) Ketogenic diets cause an increase in the HDL, or good cholesterol.

High density lipoprotein, commonly called HDL, is referred to as "good" cholesterol. However, it's actually wrong to call it cholesterol because all of the cholesterol molecules are actually the same. LDL and HDL are lipo-proteins that carry the cholesterol around within the blood.

LDL carries cholesterol from the liver to the rest of the body. HDL takes the cholesterol away from the body to the liver so that it can be processed and reused or excreted. Medical science has proven that the higher the levels of HDL in your blood, the lower your risk of developing heart disease.

Did you know that one of the best ways to increase levels of HDL in your blood is to consume more fat? Ketogenic diets contain lots of fat. Therefore, it's not at all surprising that individuals on ketogenic diets notice a dramatic increase of HDL levels.

Alternatively, the diets that focus on lower fat consumption actually cause a decrease in HDL levels.

Another strong indicator of an increased risk of heart disease is the ratio of your triglycerides to HDL. The higher this ratio is, the greater your risk for developing heart disease. Raising your HDL and lowering your triglyceride levels using a ketogenic diet will result in significant improvements in this ratio.

The Key Idea: a ketogenic diet is high in fat content, which leads to a significant increase in HDL, or "good cholesterol," levels.

6) Ketogenic diets cause lowered insulin levels and blood sugar and may significantly improve those with type 2 diabetes.

Carbohydrates break down into simple sugars, typically glucose, when entering your digestive tract. In your digestive tract, this glucose enters your blood stream and causes your blood sugar levels to rise. Since high blood sugar levels are toxic, your body will respond by producing insulin. Insulin helps gather these glucose molecules so the body can either store them or burn them.

In healthy individuals, this response happens quickly to minimize the blood sugar "spike" and protect the body.

In un-healthy individuals, there are often serious problems with this insulin system. They have what is known as **insulin resistance**. This means that the cells are unable to "see" the insulin, so it's much harder for the body to carry the glucose to the cells to store or burn them. This results in a condition known as **type 2 diabetes**.

Type 2 diabetes forms when the body doesn't produce and release enough insulin to curb the blood sugar "spike" after meals. This condition affects around 300 million people across the world today. However, there is a very simple solution to this issue: when you reduce the amount of carbohydrates you're consuming, you remove the need for the insulin. Blood sugars decrease, therefore insulin decreases.

One study showed that when put on a low-carbohydrate/ketogenic diet, 95.2 percent of diabetics were able to reduce or even eliminate their need for glucose-lowering medications within the first six months.

The bottom line is this: the best way that you can naturally lower your glucose and insulin levels is to reduce your consumption of carbohydrates. As a bonus, this is a very effective way to treat- and even reverse- type 2 diabetes.

7) Ketogenic diets cause blood pressure to decrease.

Elevated blood pressure, or hypertension, is a huge risk factor for many different conditions including: stroke, heart disease, and kidney failure, among other deadly diseases.

A ketogenic diet is an effective way to reduce blood pressure. When you reduce your blood pressure, you also reduce your risk for developing these other conditions and will live a longer, healthier, life.

The bottom line is this: studies have proven that a reduction in carbohydrate consumption causes a significant decrease in blood pressure, which will also lead to a reduced risk of developing other life-threatening conditions.

8) Ketogenic diets are the most effective treatment for metabolic syndrome.

Metabolic syndrome is a medical condition that is often associated with the risk of heart disease and diabetes. It is a combination of symptoms including the following:

A) Abdominal obesity

B) Elevated fasting blood sugar levels

C) Low HDL levels

D) High triglycerides

E) Elevated blood pressure

As we have learned, a ketogenic diet can reduce or virtually eliminate all of these symptoms. However, most major health organizations and the government still believe that a low-fat diet is best for reversing this condition, despite failing to address these underlying metabolic issues.

The bottom line is this: a ketogenic diet can reduce all five of these symptoms and eliminate the risk of metabolic syndrome.

9) A ketogenic diet will improve the pattern of LDL cholesterol.

LDL, or **low density lipo-protein**, is referred to as "bad cholesterol," but like HDL, it is actually a protein that carries the cholesterol. Science has shown that individuals with high LDL levels are much more likely to experience a heart attack than those who have low LDL levels.

However, science has now proven that not all LDL is created equal. The type of LDL that is elevated matters. This means that the size of the particles is extremely important. Those who have small particles are at an increased risk for heart disease. Those that have large particles dramatically reduce their risk for heart disease.

So how do you get larger LDL particles? A ketogenic, or low carbohydrate diet, can turn these LDL particles from small to large, as well as reduce the number of particles floating in the blood.

The bottom line is this: when consuming a ketogenic diet, the LDL particles in your blood will change from small to large. Additionally, cutting carbohydrate consumption will reduce the number of particles floating in your blood.

10) Ketogenic diets are therapeutic for several different disorders of the brain.

You often hear that glucose is a necessity for functioning of the brain- and this is true. There are some parts of your brain that can only burn glucose. This is why your liver makes glucose from proteins if we're not consuming any carbohydrates.

Additionally, a large portion of the brain can also burn ketones. These are formed during starvation or when your consumption of carbohydrates is low. This is how the ketogenic diet works. Your brain will transition from burning glucose to burning ketones. In some individuals, this switch can give them clearer thinking and eliminate "brain fog." By clearing up your brain, you will feel better, have more energy, and be more productive, while also eliminating your risk for several brain diseases.

Ketogenic diets are currently being studied as treatments for other brain disorders including Parkinson's and Alzheimer's.

Chapter 4
Understanding the Basics of Ketogenic Nutrition

According to research, the ketogenic diet is an extreme version of the many low carbohydrate diets. However, its results in treating conditions like pediatric epilepsy and assisting in tumor regression is increasingly becoming a topic of study among researchers across the world.

The definition of a ketogenic diet is one that is low in carbohydrates, high in fats, and moderate in proteins. Some individuals have followed a ketogenic diet for weight loss and have reported short-term success after several months by consuming high fat, low carbohydrate meals every day. Additionally, other studies have revealed some beneficial side effects of this diet including a reduction in bad cholesterol and an increase in good cholesterol. However, though this diet can cause rapid weight loss, it is vital that you consult a physician before beginning this, or any other, diet plan.

How does the ketogenic diet work?

The ketogenic diet works by shifting the body's energy source to fats instead of carbohydrates. When your body has entered what is known as a fasting state, it creates molecules that are known as ketone bodies. These build up as your body is burning fat for energy- and the process is known as ketosis.

The reason this happens is not really clear. However, researchers do believe that the increase in ketone bodies within the blood can reduce or reverse many diseases.

What are the characteristics of the Ketogenic Diet?

Basically, the ratio of carbohydrates to fats and proteins is 1:4. Of course, it is necessary to tailor this ratio for each individual. A typical range would involve the individual consuming approximately 60 percent of their calories from fats, 35 percent of their calories from proteins, and only 5 percent of their calories from carbohydrates.

When you're just starting out, it is highly recommended that you limit your carbohydrate consumption to about 20 grams each day so that your body can enter a state of ketosis. Once you have done so, you can start increasing your carbohydrate intake to around 50 grams per day- but no more. This is reflective of the amount of carbohydrates that your body can use in one day. Of course, these numbers are not concrete, but are dependent upon the metabolism and activity level of each individual. In order to accurately track the amount of fats, proteins, and carbohydrates you are consuming, it is highly recommended you invest in a kitchen scale and an application to track your calories. I would highly recommend using the free app called MyFitnessPal and the scale that is in my Amazon store @ http://amzn.to/1KfzSWS

Some people can find this type of diet hard to follow since it can limit the variety and the types of food allowed. You will be eating mostly proteins, veggies (especially green leafy ones), and fats that make up most of the calories in your diet. If you are consistently eating the same foods over and over, you may eventually become deficient in certain vitamins and minerals.
If you want to achieve success on a ketogenic diet, you must be willing to completely follow and be fully committed to making it work for you.

Following are some tips on what to eat and what not to eat - as well as some general ketogenic diet tips.

Foods that You Can Eat

Choose plenty of green leafy veggies such as broccoli, cabbage, cauliflower, celery, cucumbers, lettuce, and spinach. You must limit your consumption of tomatoes, onions, red and yellow peppers, and starchy veggies such as potatoes because these contain high levels of carbohydrates.

When you feel like you need a snack, choose boiled eggs, cheese, or peanut butter. You can consume moderate amounts of nuts, but watch out for almonds, walnuts, cashews, and macadamias, as these have higher levels of carbohydrates.

You can cut and prepare meat such as lamb, beef, or pork any way that you choose.

When preparing poultry, leave the skin on in order to increase the fat content. You can also prepare this any way that you choose.

Foods that Should Be Avoided

Avoid consuming low-fat foods, since all of your calories and energy are coming from fat. You want to make sure you're eating products that are high in fat such as bacon, full-fat dairy, and other healthy fats.

When drinking coffee, you should avoid adding extra milk and sugar and instead opt for a natural sweetener and replace milk with heavy cream or almond milk for an alternative that is low in carbohydrates.

Never choose fruits as a snack, whether frozen, dried, or fresh because they are very high in carbohydrates and fructose. If you must have something sweet, choose a lower-carb food like strawberries. However, you should be aware that the fructose may prevent your body from entering ketosis, so it may be best to avoid them completely.

You should avoid grain and grain products, fruit and high-sugar veggie juices, 1 percent or skim milk, lentils, beer, and beans, which are all very high in carbohydrate levels.

Important Tips to Keep in Mind

When choosing foods, make sure that you check the carbohydrate content of every single thing you plan to eat. Some foods contain hidden carbohydrates. For example, you may have a low carbohydrate mustard, but added sweeteners and/or honey can cause the level of carbohydrates to increase. You also want to make sure you double check the carbohydrate content of oil-based salad dressings and mayonnaise. For a full-list of foods that are safe to eat, refer to the grocery list download at the beginning of this book.

Again, make sure that you're keeping track of your food/carbohydrate consumption. You can keep it on a spreadsheet on your computer, in an online food tracker like MyFitnessPal, or even keep them recorded in a journal. Also, take the time to reflect and write down how you're feeling each day as well as any changes you made in your diet or life. This way, if you do get off track, you can figure out where you went wrong and get yourself realigned. This will also keep you motivated throughout your journey.

Make sure you consistently choose the low carbohydrate options so that you avoid exceeding your daily limit. Additionally, make sure to check labels for net carbohydrates- which you can calculate by taking the total carbs and subtracting the amount of fiber.

It's also recommended you take a multivitamin in order to replenish the vitamins and minerals you may not be ingesting.

Chapter 5
5 Mistakes to Avoid on a Ketogenic Diet

According to Dr. Jeff S. Volek, a registered dietician, and Dr. Stephen D. Phinney, a medical doctor, there are several stumbling blocks that people often run into when it comes to ketogenic/low carbohydrate diets. These two physicians have done many studies and treated thousands of patients with ketogenic diets. They state that these stumbling blocks can cause adverse effects as well as sub-optimal results.

In order to get to a full-blown ketosis state and get all of the metabolic benefits of a low carbohydrate lifestyle, there is much more to it than simply cutting back on carbohydrate consumption.

This chapter will provide 5 of the most common mistakes that people make when adopting a ketogenic diet - as well as how to avoid them.

1) Individuals often consume too many carbohydrates.

The definition of "low carb diet" is not really all that clear. Some individuals would say that anything under 100 to 150 grams of carbohydrates per day would be considered low carb as this is most definitely less than what the average person consumes in a traditional Western diet.

Most people would be able to get excellent results within this range, as long as they were consuming unprocessed, real foods. However, if you want to achieve full ketosis, with lots of ketones flowing through your bloodstream and supplying your brain with energy, this is probably too many carbohydrates.

While it will most likely take some self-experimentation to figure out your personal optimal range, most people will need under 50 grams of carbohydrates each day to reach full ketosis.

The bottom line is this: if you wish to reach full ketosis and reap all the metabolic benefits of a low-carbohydrate lifestyle, you must consume less than 50 grams of carbohydrates daily.

2) Individuals often consume too much protein.

Of course, you know that protein is an extremely vital macronutrient, and most people do not get enough of it. Compared to other macronutrients, protein can increase fat burning and improve satiety.

Overall, consuming more protein should result in weight loss and an improvement in body composition. However, in many cases, individuals on a ketogenic diet actually end up eating too many lean animal foods and consuming excess amounts of protein.

When you consume more protein than your body requires, some of the amino acids in the proteins will turn into glucose through **gluconeogenesis**. This becomes a problem because it keeps your body from entering complete ketosis. According to Phinney and Volek, a ketogenic diet should be a combination of low-carbohydrate, moderate protein, and high fat. The best range to aim for is 1.5 to 2.0 grams of protein per kilogram of body weight or 0.7 to 0.9 grams of protein per pound of bodyweight.

The bottom line is this: excessive levels of protein will be turned into glucose through gluconeogenesis and will keep your body from entering ketosis.

3) Individuals are often afraid of consuming fats.

Traditionally, most people get the main part of their daily calories from carbohydrates, especially grains and sugars. Therefore, when you take out this energy source, you must find something else to replace it with so that you do not starve. The bad part about it is that most people think that since low carbohydrate diets are a good idea that low-fat/low carbohydrate will be so much better. However, this is a huge mistake.

You must get your energy from somewhere and if you're not eating carbohydrates, then you've got to add some fat in your diet in order to compensate. If you don't do this, you'll end up getting hungry, feeling terrible, and will ultimately give up on your plan.

There is no reason that you should fear fats, as long as you're choosing healthy fats such as omega-3s, saturated, and monounsaturated. You must consume minimal amounts of vegetable oils and eliminate trans fats from your diet.

Personally, when I'm sticking to a ketogenic, or other low carbohydrate, diet my fat intake is about 50 to 60 percent of my total caloric intake. According to Phinney and Volek, an intake of around 70 percent of calories from fat is ideal.

In order to bring your fat intake into this range, you must select fatty cuts of meat and add lots of healthy fats such as olive oil, grass-fed butter, and coconut oil to your meals.

The bottom line is this: when you are on a ketogenic diet, you must increase your fat intake to be the majority of your caloric intake or you will feel miserable.

4) Individuals often don't replenish sodium.

One of the main functions behind the low-carbohydrate diet is the reduction in the levels of insulin- which has many functions within the body. Insulin is what tells your body's fat cells to store fat. Additionally, insulin tells your kidneys to hold on to the sodium in your body.

Sodium is important. When you're on a ketogenic diet, your insulin levels decrease, which causes your body to shed excess water and sodium. This is the reason why people typically rid themselves of excess bloat within just a few days of beginning any type of low-carbohydrate diet.

However, something you should know is that sodium is a critical electrolyte in your body and losing it becomes an issue when your kidneys are dumping lots of it. This is why lots of people develop side-effects such as fatigue, constipation, lightheadedness, and even headaches when on a ketogenic diet. It is also the reason that athletes experience cramps and other negative symptoms when they do not consume enough sodium.

The best way to avoid these uncomfortable side effects is to add additional sodium to your diet. Of course, this can be done by adding more salt to your foods or by drinking a cup of broth each day.

My favorite thing to do is add one bouillon cube to a cup of hot water and drink it like soup. Believe it or not, it tastes pretty good and gives me two grams of sodium.

The bottom line is this: when you're on a ketogenic diet, your insulin levels will be reduced, making the kidneys excrete excess water and sodium from the body. Ensure you are consuming enough sodium to keep you functioning at your best.

5) Individuals are often not patient enough.

Your body is made to burn carbohydrates when they are available. Therefore, when you're always consuming carbs, your body will be burning them for energy. However, when you drastically reduce your consumption of them, your body will shift to a different energy source - fat in your diet or fat stored in your body.

Of course, it's going to take a few days for your body to get used to burning fat instead of carbohydrates. You'll likely feel a little under-the-weather during this time. Most people who are switching to a ketogenic diet feel this way and it is referred to as the "low-carb flu."

In my personal experience, this typically takes three to four days. However, your body may take up to several weeks to fully adapt to this new lifestyle. It is critical that you are very strict in sticking with the diet in the beginning so that your body has the time it needs to process this metabolic adaptation.

The bottom line is this: it will likely take you a few days to get over this "low carb flu" and your body may take several weeks to fully adjust. Therefore, you must be very disciplined and patient and think of the ketogenic diet as a lifestyle and not another diet.

Part Two

Getting Started with the Ketogenic Diet

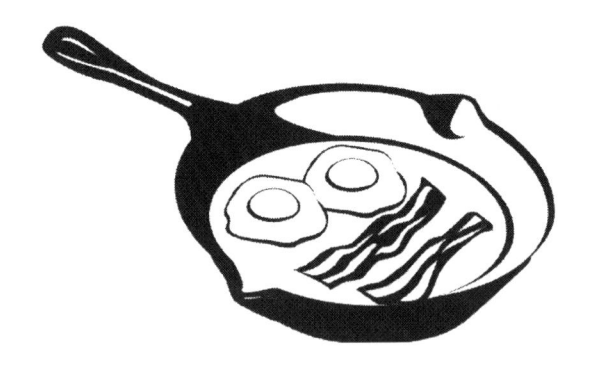

Chapter 6
11 Tips for Getting Started on a Ketogenic Diet

Now that you know all about the ketogenic diet, you must learn a few tips for beginning your journey:

1) It's recommended you keep your carbohydrates under 50, preferably 20, grams per day. After all, that's what keto is all about. Count every single carb that you eat. I would highly suggest using the free app, MyFitnessPal. MyFitnessPal allows you to scan the barcode of foods you eat and allows you to easily and conveniently track your calories and weight-loss. You can also access the app and your account from your computer or phone.

2) 65 percent of your calories should come from fats, 30 percent from proteins, and only 5 percent from carbs. If you're not sure how to balance this out, check out some of the online fitness sites or smartphone apps. Again, MyFitnessPal makes this very easy to do.

3) Avoid excess protein: consuming too much protein will result in an increase in insulin levels, and therefore, will reduce your weight-loss progress.

4) Don't allow yourself any cheat days - it's not worth it.

5) Make sure you stay hydrated by drinking plenty of water. This diet will flush out your system, so you want to be mindful about rehydrating. I aim for 1 gallon per day. You may benefit from picking up a few gallons of water from the store to ensure you always have water available.

6) For the first two to three weeks, you can drink one cup of chicken broth each day. After all, when water is flushed from your system, so are your electrolytes. Broth is a great way to bring your salt levels back up to a healthy range. Invest in some bouillon cubes for convenience.

7) Unless you are used to exercise and your body can handle it, don't do any high-intensity exercise for the first two to three weeks. Your body will be going through enough changes and you want to limit the additional stress. If you want to remain active, schedule walks and light cardio or weight-training into your daily routine.

8) You're going to want to do a body comparison, so make sure that you take pictures of your body from all sides when you're getting started. I'd also recommend taking updated progress pictures every 1-2 weeks so you can see your progress. Include your current weight with these pictures and an update on how you are feeling both mentally and physically.

9) Understand that there is a difference between ketoacidosis and ketosis. There are lots of misconceptions about this and it's a good idea to make sure you educate yourself so that you can respond correctly when someone tells you that ketosis is dangerous.

10) Every day, aim to find something professionally published regarding keto, nutrition, low carb, etc. to read and learn more about the keto way of life. Gaining more knowledge will help keep you motivated and on track to reaching your goals.

11) Always remain respectful of diets/lifestyles of others who may not believe the way you do- but also make sure you know and can explain why you are living a ketogenic lifestyle. Knowing this before you get started will ensure that you stick to it, especially under adversity.

Chapter 7
Grocery Lists and Foods You Should Be Eating

If you're just getting started on a keto diet, chances are you might not know what to buy at the grocery store. Following is a list of the most popular and tasty ketogenic foods, listed according to category. Make sure to **download the free printable grocery list @ http://bit.ly/1V24Kjf**

Grocery List For Keto Shopping

Meats/Proteins
- Bacon
- Ground Beef
- Steak
- Pork or Beef Ribs
- Pork or Beef Roasts
- Pork Loin, Pork Steaks, Pork Chops
- Chicken
- Sausage
- Ham
- Deli Meats
- Salami
- Prosciutto
- Eggs

Seafood/Fish
- Cod
- Scallops
- Shrimp
- Crab
- Tilapia
- Albacore
- Tuna
- Salmon

Dairy
- Sour Cream
- Cheese
- Butter
- Heavy Cream
- Cream Cheese

Other
- Unsweetened Almond Milk
- Unsweetened Cocoa Powder
- Pickles
- Olives
- Herbs/Spices
- Olive Oil/Coconut Oil
- Beef Jerky
- Pork Rinds

Chapter 8
15 Super-Convenient Breakfast Recipes

You want to get your day started off right - so here are 15 super-easy and convenient keto breakfast ideas and recipes. Make sure to **download these free recipe cards @ http://bit.ly/1V24Kjf**

1. Quick-n-Easy Ketogenic Breakfast Mix

Ingredients
- ✓ *5 TBSP unsweetened coconut flakes*
- ✓ *2 TBSP ground sesame*
- ✓ *5 TBSP ground flaxseed*
- ✓ *2 TBSP unsweetened dark cocoa*
- ✓ *7 TBSP hemp seeds*

1) Grind together the sesame and the flax. Be sure that you only grind the sesame seeds enough to crack them- otherwise, you'll have a paste.

2) Combine all ingredients in a jar and shake. You will end up with 23 TBSP of this mix.

3) The hemp and sesame seeds are very high in fat, so you'll need to keep this in the fridge.

4) You can serve with black coffee or water. Add coconut oil if you want to increase the fat content. This also blends quite well with mascarpone cheese or cream. If you wish, add liquid sweetener or stevia.

2. Creamy Ricotta and Eggs

Ingredients
- ✓ 2 whole eggs
- ✓ 1 TBSP olive oil
- ✓ 50 grams Italian dry salami
- ✓ 150 grams 2% fat ricotta cheese
- ✓ 1 tsp rosemary
- ✓ Salt/Pepper to taste

1) Chop salami into cubes and pan fry with olive oil.
2) Whisk eggs, add rosemary, salt, and pepper.
3) Add the ricotta into the eggs, mixing well with a fork, breaking down the large lumps.
4) Add ricotta and eggs, cooking until done - about 5 minutes. Serve hot. I LOVE this recipe and often eat it for lunch and dinner.

3. Hardboiled Buttery Eggs

Ingredients
- ✓ *2 whole eggs*
- ✓ *1 TBSP mascarpone cheese*
- ✓ *30 grams butter*
- ✓ *Salt/Pepper to taste*

1) Hard boil eggs with a pinch of salt - this helps eggs to peel once done.
2) Wash eggs with cold water quickly. Then peel and chop them.
3) Add mascarpone cheese and butter while eggs are hot, mixing well. Add salt/pepper to taste.

4. Coconut and Coffee Cup

Ingredients
- ✓ *30 grams flaxseed*
- ✓ *1 TBSP coconut oil*
- ✓ *½ cup unsweetened black coffee*
- ✓ *30 grams unsweetened coconut flakes*
- ✓ *Liquid sweetener if desired*

1) Mix together coconut flakes and flax in bowl.
2) Add coconut oil.
3) Pour over coffee and mix. You can adjust thickness by adding more mix or more coffee or water.
4) Add sweetener if desired.

5. Fried Cheddar Slices

Ingredients
- ✓ 2 slices cheddar cheese
- ✓ 1 tsp ground flaxseed
- ✓ 1 tsp hemp
- ✓ 1 whole egg
- ✓ 1 TBSP olive oil
- ✓ 1 tsp almond flour
- ✓ Salt/pepper to taste

1) Heat olive oil in pan on medium heat.
2) Whisk egg with salt and pepper in bowl.
3) Mix ground flax with hemp and almond flour in separate bowl.
4) Coat cheddar with egg mix then dry mix. Fry for approximately three minutes.

6. Sweet Vanilla Ricotta Cheese

Ingredients
- ✓ 200 grams 2% fat ricotta cheese
- ✓ 1 TBSP crème fraiche
- ✓ 1 sachet vanilla flavor

1) Mix together ricotta cheese, crème fraiche, and vanilla in bowl. If you prefer, make your own vanilla flavor by scraping pulp off of a vanilla pod and mix it with liquid sweetener. This recipe tastes like dessert to me!

7. Cream, Flax, and Goji Cereal

Ingredients

- ✓ *100 ml cooking cream*
- ✓ *1 tsp dark unsweetened cocoa powder*
- ✓ *1 TBSP Goji berries*
- ✓ *30 grams ground flaxseed*
- ✓ *Fresh brewed coffee*
- ✓ *Liquid sweetener*

1) Mix ground flax and cocoa with cream until covered. Add liquid sweetener if desired.

2) Add just a little coffee- the flax will expand quite a bit. If you don't care for coffee, you can substitute hot water. Rooibos or black tea are also great options to soften the flax.

3) Decorate with the berries and enjoy!

8. Delicious Deli Rolls

Ingredients
- ✓ *8 ounces full fat cream cheese*
- ✓ *Quality deli meats*

1) Place deli meats between clean paper towels and dry them.

2) Bring cream cheese to room temperature.

3) Spread thin layer of cream cheese on slices of meat and roll up. Repeat until you use up the deli meat. Chill overnight.

9. Overnight Greek Yogurt & Protein Cups

Ingredients
- ✓ *6 ounces full fat, unsweetened Greek yogurt*
- ✓ *½ scoop unsweetened whey protein powder*
- ✓ *1 ounce heavy cream*

1) Mix all ingredients well.

2) Refrigerate overnight. Make a few at a time - that way you always have them on hand and can grab them and go.

10. Keto Breakfast Pizza
Ingredients

- ✓ *4 large eggs*
- ✓ *3 TBSP almond flour*
- ✓ *1 tsp baking powder*
- ✓ *4 TBSP Parmesan cheese*
- ✓ *1 TBSP psyllium powder*
- ✓ *1 tsp Italian seasoning (or spices of your choice)*
- ✓ *1 TBSP butter or bacon grease*
- ✓ *3 ounce cheddar cheese*
- ✓ *½ cup tomato sauce*
- ✓ *14 slices pepperoni, if desired*
- ✓ *Salt/pepper to taste*

1) Combine all ingredients in a bowl, except cheese and tomato sauce.

2) Blend everything together using an immersion blender- approximately thirty to forty-five seconds until thick.

3) Heat waffle iron (or hot pan) and add half of mixture.

4) Allow to cook until steam rises from waffle iron. Once done, remove and repeat.

5) Add tomato sauce, cheese, and pepperoni (if desired) to the top and broil for three to five minutes in oven.

6) Once cheese is melted, remove from oven and serve.

11. Breakfast Keto Burger
Ingredients

- ✓ *2 ounce pepper jack cheese*
- ✓ *4 ounce sausage*
- ✓ *2 large eggs*
- ✓ *4 slices bacon*
- ✓ *1 TBSP dehydrated peanut butter powder*
- ✓ *1 TBSP butter*
- ✓ *Salt/Pepper to taste*

1) Cook bacon by laying strips on a wire rack over a cookie sheet. Bake at 400 degrees for about 20-25 minutes or until preferred crispness.

2) Mix together butter and peanut butter powder in a small container and set aside.

3) Form sausage into two patties and cook them over medium-high heat in frying pan. Flip when bottom side is browned.

4) Grate cheese and set aside.

5) Once second side of sausage is brown, top with cheese and cover with lid.

6) Remove sausage and set aside. Fry egg in the same pan.

7) Assemble everything and top with rehydrated peanut butter. Enjoy!

12. Cheesy Bacon, Cheddar, and Chive Omelette
Ingredients
- ✓ *1 tsp bacon grease*
- ✓ *1 ounce cheddar cheese*
- ✓ *2 slices already cooked bacon*
- ✓ *2 large eggs*
- ✓ *2 chive stalks*
- ✓ *Salt/pepper to taste*

1) Precook bacon, shred cheese and chop chives before starting because the omelette will cook quickly.

2) Heat pan with bacon fat over medium-low heat. When you hold your hand above the pan, you should be able to feel a decent amount of heat from it. Add in the eggs and chives and season with salt and pepper if desired.

3) Once edges set, add bacon, cover, and allow to cook for twenty to thirty seconds, then turn off heat.

4) Add cheese and then fold over two edges of the omelette on top of the cheese. Hold for a moment so the cheese acts as a "glue" to hold them.

5) Do the same with other edges, creating a burrito. Flip and allow to cook in the warm pan for a little bit longer.

6) Serve with extra bacon, chives, and cheese if you wish.

13. Leftover Meat Sampler
Cold meats from the previous evening's dinner make a yummy, quick breakfast. Throw in an ounce of hard cheese and/or macadamia nuts to round it out.

14. Low Carb Muffins
Make low-carbohydrate muffins using your favorite muffin recipe but use almond flour instead of regular flour and a zero-calorie sweetener. Under 6 grams of carbohydrates each. These are especially good when you add butter.

15. Quick Protein Shake
The only thing you need for this is a blender bottle, unsweetened almond milk, and some low-carb protein powder. Simply pour 8-16 ounces of milk in the blender bottle, add protein powder, shake it up and enjoy!

Chapter 9
Top 15 Lunch-On-The-Go Recipes

When it comes to lunches, it's much better to make them at home and take them with you than to trust that you can find takeout that works with your keto diet. Here are 15 super-easy keto lunch ideas. You can make most of these ahead of time so that you can just grab and go. Make sure to **download these free recipe cards @ http://bit.ly/1V24Kjf**

1. ABC Sandwich (Avocado, Bacon, and Chicken)
Ingredients
Keto Bread
- ✓ 3 large eggs
- ✓ 1/8 tsp cream of tartar
- ✓ 1/2 tsp garlic powder
- ✓ 1/4 tsp salt
- ✓ 3 ounces cream cheese

Filling
- ✓ 2 slices bacon
- ✓ 1 TBSP Mayo
- ✓ 1 tsp sriracha sauce
- ✓ 2 slices pepper jack
- ✓ 3 ounces chicken
- ✓ 1/4 medium avocado
- ✓ 2 grape tomatoes

1) Preheat oven to 300 degrees. Separate 3 eggs into two clean and dry bowls. One bowl for the yolks and one for the whites.

2) Add cream of tartar and salt to egg whites and whip with electric mixer until you create soft, foamy peaks.

3) In the bowl with yolks, combine cream cheese, beating until a pale yellow.

4) Gently fold whites into yolk mixture half at a time.

5) On parchment paper, spoon approximately ¼ cup of the batter. You'll get six large pieces of bread.

6) Using a spatula, press gently on tops of batter to make squares. Sprinkle with garlic powder and bake for 25 minutes.

7) While bread is baking, cook chicken and bacon with salt and pepper.

8) Combine mayo and sriracha sauce and spread on the underside of a slice of keto bread. Add chicken to mayo mixture.

9) Add 2 slices of cheese and bacon, some halved grape tomatoes, spread avocado on top. Season it to your liking and top with another piece of keto bread.

2. Fresh Caesar Salad

Ingredients

- ✓ 1 egg yolk
- ✓ 3 TBSP apple cider vinegar
- ✓ 4 anchovy filets
- ✓ 8 TBSP avocado oil
- ✓ 4 TBSP grated parmesan
- ✓ 1 tsp Dijon mustard
- ✓ 2 ounces pork rinds, crumbled
- ✓ 24 whole romaine leaves
- ✓ 4 TBSP shaved parmesan

1) In an immersion blender, combine egg yolk, apple cider vinegar, and mustard. Place blender stick on yolk and carefully pour avocado oil on top.

2) Start blender on low, but don't move stick from its current position.

3) Egg yolk should emulsify with oil and create a mayo mixture.

4) Once ready, remove blender and add in the anchovy filets, grated parmesan, and garlic.

5) Blend slowly until well-blended to create a smooth mayo dressing.

6) Wash and dry romaine leaves and separate into four serving plates.

7) Drizzle dressing on leaves.

8) Divide crumbled pork rinds and garnish with shaved parmesan.

3. Salmon and Avocado Sushi
Ingredients
- ✓ 500 grams cauli-rice
- ✓ 1 TBSP rice vinegar
- ✓ 50 grams smoked salmon
- ✓ 2 TBSP softened butter
- ✓ Whipped cream cheese
- ✓ 1 sliced avocado
- ✓ 4 nori papers

1) On medium heat, add cauli-rice to butter and saute for ten to fifteen minutes. Allow to rest until cool.

2) While cauli-rice is cooling, coat nori papers with a layer of cream cheese.

3) Add rice vinegar to cauli-rice and stir.

4) Pat rice mixture onto the cream cheese in a thin layer.

5) On the edge of the paper, place salmon and avocado pieces. Roll up and enjoy!

4. Low-Carb Lunch Pizza
Ingredients
Crust
- ✓ 1 cup chia seeds
- ✓ 1 tsp celtic sea salt
- ✓ 1 cup water
- ✓ 1 medium cauliflower
- ✓ 3 TBSP olive oil

Keto Topping
- ✓ 1/2 cup grated parmesan
- ✓ 1/2 cup heavy cream
- ✓ 1/2 cup cream cheese
- ✓ 2 peeled garlic cloves

Crust

1) Remove cauliflower florets and finely chop them.
2) Grind chia seeds into a flour.
3) Mix chia, salt, cauliflower, olive oil and water, mixing until a smooth dough is formed.
4) Allow to rest for twenty minutes.
5) Spread olive oil on a cookie sheet. Spread dough about 1/2 inch thick, or if preferred, use two cookie sheets and spread thinner.
6) Bake at 100 degrees for around one hour, or until crust is cooked and dry. Depending upon thickness, time could vary.
7) Once crust is done, raise temp to 400 degrees.

Topping

8) Mix cheeses, garlic, and cream until you create a paste.

9) Spread on crust and bake at 400 degrees for approximately ten minutes. Enjoy!

5. Mixed Green Spring Salad

Ingredients

- ✓ *2 ounce mixed greens*
- ✓ *2 TBSP Raspberry Vinaigrette*
- ✓ *3 TBSP roasted pine nuts*
- ✓ *2 slices bacon*
- ✓ *2 TBSP shaved parmesan*
- ✓ *Salt/Pepper to taste*

   1) *Cook bacon until crisp. Allow to cool, then crumble.*

   2) *Measure out greens and set in a container that you can shake.*

   3) *Add bacon and remaining ingredients to greens. Shake and enjoy!*

6. Cheesy Bacon Wrapped Hot Dogs

Ingredients
- ✓ *6 hot dogs*
- ✓ *12 bacon slices*
- ✓ *1/2 tsp each garlic powder and onion powder*
- ✓ *2 ounces cheddar cheese*
- ✓ *Salt/pepper to taste*

1) Preheat oven to 400 degrees.
2) Slit all of the hot dogs down the middle.
3) Slice cheese into small, long rectangles and stuff into hot dogs.
4) Tightly wrap one slice of bacon around hot dog. Take a second slice and slightly overlapping the first one, continue wrapping.
5) Poke toothpicks in each side of bacon/hot dog to secure bacon in place.
6) Place on a wire rack on top of a cookie sheet and season with salt, pepper, onion powder, and garlic powder.
7) Bake for thirty-five to forty minutes until bacon is crisp. If desired, broil bacon on top.

7. Egg Drop Soup
Ingredients

- ✓ 1 1/2 cup chicken broth
- ✓ 1 TBSP butter or bacon fat
- ✓ 1/2 cube chicken bullion
- ✓ 1 tsp chili garlic paste
- ✓ 2 large eggs

1) Place pan on stove and heat to medium high. Then, add chicken broth, bullion and the butter or bacon fat.

2) Bring broth to a boil, stirring everything together. Add chili garlic paste and stir. Turn off stove.

3) Beat eggs in a separate bowl, then pour into broth mixture.

4) Stir together well, and allow to sit for 1 minute to finish cooking.

Sausage and Pepper Soup
Ingredients

- ✓ 32 ounce sausage
- ✓ 10 ounce spinach, raw
- ✓ 1 can tomatoes/jalapenos
- ✓ 1 TBSP olive oil
- ✓ 1 medium green pepper
- ✓ 1 TBSP chili powder
- ✓ 1 tsp garlic powder
- ✓ 4 cups beef stock
- ✓ 1 tsp onion powder
- ✓ 1 TBSP cumin
- ✓ 3/4 tsp kosher salt
- ✓ 1 tsp Italian seasoning

1) Heat olive oil in pot over medium heat. When hot, add sausage.

2) When sausage is seared on bottom, mix the sausage together to allow it to cook thoroughly.

3) While sausage is cooking, slice green pepper. Add peppers to sausage and mix together well. Season with salt/pepper.

4) Add tomatoes/jalapenos and stir one more time.

5) Add spinach on top and place lid on pot, cooking for 6-7 minutes or until spinach is wilted.

6) While cooking, measure out the spices and get the beef stock ready.

7) *When the spinach is wilted, mix it with the sausage. Then add the spices and mix once more. Finally, add broth and mix again.*

8) *Reduce heat and replace lid, cooking for 30 minutes.*

9) *Remove lid and simmer for 15 more minutes.*

Buffalo Chicken Crockpot Soup
Ingredients

- ✓ 3 medium deboned, sliced chicken thighs
- ✓ 1 tsp each garlic and onion powder
- ✓ 1/4 cup butter
- ✓ 1/2 tsp celery seed
- ✓ 1/3 to 1/2 cup hot sauce, depending on preference
- ✓ 3 ounce cream cheese
- ✓ 3 cups beef broth
- ✓ 1 cup heavy cream
- ✓ Salt/pepper to taste

1) Debone and slice/cube chicken thighs, dropping them into crockpot.

2) Add remainder of ingredients except cream and cheese. Set on low for 6 hours or high for 3 hours.

3) Once everything is cooked, remove chicken and shred with a fork.

4) Add cream and cheese to crockpot. Use an immersion blender and emulsify all liquids together.

5) Place chicken back into crockpot and stir. Season to taste with salt, pepper, and hot sauce if desired.

10. Magic Meat Muffins

Ingredients

- ✓ 1/2 pound cleaned mushrooms
- ✓ 1 pound ground beef
- ✓ 1 tsp sea salt
- ✓ 6 egg yolks
- ✓ 3/4 cup coconut flour

1) Preheat oven to 350 degrees.

2) In food processor, roughly chop mushrooms, add egg yolk, and salt and process until smooth.

3) Transfer mixture to a large bowl and add ground beef, mixing well.

4) Add coconut flour, using a sifter to avoid clumping.

5) You should have a soft and pliable dough that is firm enough to make a meatball.

6) Place 13 paper cupcake cups on a cookie sheet or muffin pan and make 13 meatballs to place inside them.

7) Place in oven and bake for forty-five minutes or until brown on top and moist inside.

8) These can be enjoyed hot or cold.

11. Pesto Chicken Salad

<u>Ingredients</u>

- ✓ *1 pound cubed and cooked chicken*
- ✓ *1 cubed avocado*
- ✓ *6 slices cooked, crisp, crumbled bacon*
- ✓ *10 halved grape tomatoes*
- ✓ *2 TBSP garlic pesto*
- ✓ *1/4 cup mayo*
- ✓ *Fresh butter lettuce leaves*

1) (This one is really simple) In a large bowl, mix together all ingredients and enjoy!

12. Chimichurri and Steak Salad

Ingredients

- ✓ 1/3 cup shredded red cabbage
- ✓ 2 cup shredded romaine hearts
- ✓ 2 TBSP fresh cilantro
- ✓ 3 thinly sliced radishes
- ✓ 3 TBSP chimichurri sauce
- ✓ 1 TBSP vinaigrette salad dressing
- ✓ 4 ounces steak
- ✓ 1 ounce blue cheese, if desired

1) Toss together the romaine, cilantro, red cabbage, and radish with vinaigrette.

2) Serve steak, thinly sliced on the side with chimichurri sauce for dipping.

3) If desired, add blue cheese crumbles to top.

13. Microwave Keto Grilled Cheese

Ingredients

Bread

- ✓ *2 TBSP almond flour*
- ✓ *1 1/2 TBSP psyllium powder*
- ✓ *2 TBSP soft butter*
- ✓ *2 large eggs*
- ✓ *1/2 tsp baking powder*

Filling/Extras

- ✓ *1 TBSP butter*
- ✓ *2 ounces cheddar cheese (or preferred cheese)*

1) Allow butter to soften to room temperature in a mug. Once soft, add almond flour, psyllium, and baking powder.

2) Mix together to form a thick dough.

3) Add eggs and continue mixing. You want your dough to be thick. If not thick enough, keep mixing, it will thicken as you mix and may take up to 1 minute.

4) Pour dough into square bowl or container and level off.

5) Microwave for approximately 90-100 seconds. If not cooked, add another 20-30 seconds.

6) Remove by flipping upside down and tapping the bottom of the mug. Then, cut in half with bread knife.

7) Measure cheese and place between pieces of bread.

8) Heat 1 TBSP butter in a pan over medium heat. When hot, add bread and allow to cook in butter. Butter will be absorbed, giving the bread a crisp outside. Enjoy!

14. Caprese Salad

Ingredients

- ¼ cup chopped fresh basil
- 1 fresh tomato
- Fresh cracked black pepper
- Kosher salt
- 6 ounce fresh mozzarella cheese
- 3 TBSP olive oil

1) First make the basil paste by pulsing chopped basil leaves with 2 TBSP olive oil.

2) Slice tomato in 1/4 inch slices- you should get 6 slices from one tomato.

3) Cut mozzarella in 1 ounce slices.

4) Assemble by layering tomato, mozzarella, and topping with basil paste.

5) Season with salt, pepper, and left over olive oil.

15. Walnut and Fennel Chicken Salad

Ingredients

- ✓ 3 cooked boneless, skinless chicken breasts
- ✓ 1/4 cup toasted, chopped walnuts
- ✓ 1 1/2 cup coarsely chopped fennel
- ✓ 2 TBSP walnut oil
- ✓ 2 TBSP fennel fronds, chopped
- ✓ 1/4 cup mayo
- ✓ 2 TBSP fresh squeezed lemon juice
- ✓ 2 pressed garlic cloves
- ✓ 1/8 tsp cayenne pepper
- ✓ Salt/Pepper to taste

1) Toss cooked chicken, walnuts, and fennel in large bowl until combined.

2) Whisk together mayo, lemon juice, garlic, cayenne, walnut oil, lemon juice, and chopped fennel fronds until smooth.

3) Pour dressing mixture over chicken and toss. Season with salt/pepper if desired. Allow to chill for at least 1 hour in fridge. The longer you allow it to sit, the more it will bring out the flavors.

Chapter 10

Top 15 Delicious Dinner Recipes

It's the end of the day and all you want are some quick and easy dinner recipes to keep you on your keto track. Here are 15 great-tasting recipes. **download these free recipe cards @ http://bit.ly/1V24Kjf**

1) Garlic Lebanese Chicken

Ingredients
- 2 TBSP ghee
- 1 vidalia onion, quartered
- Garlic olive oil
- 4 chicken thighs
- 2 roma tomatoes, halved
- Oregano
- 15 whole garlic cloves
- Handful of baby carrots
- Juice from one fresh lemon
- Salt/pepper to taste

1) Heat oven to 500 degrees and glaze bottom of cast-iron pan with 2 TBSP of garlic olive oil.
2) Add chicken thighs, leaving space between them.
3) Between thighs, wedge onions, garlic, tomatoes, and carrots. Add 1-2 garlic cloves on top of each thigh. Juice lemon over top.

4) Drizzle garlic oil and ghee over top of thighs.

5) Sprinkle oregano generously and salt/pepper to taste.

6) Place in oven for 30 minutes.

7) Reduce oven to 350 degrees and cook for another 20 minutes or until chicken is 165 degrees when measured with meat thermometer.

8) Increase to broil and cook for 5 minutes or until crisp.

2) Keto Chicken Parmesan and Zoodles

Ingredients
- ✓ 2 cups pork rinds, crushed
- ✓ 4 chicken breasts, pounded and tenderized
- ✓ 4 medium zucchinis
- ✓ 1 cup parmesan cheese, grated
- ✓ 2 TBSP Italian seasoning
- ✓ 1 tsp garlic salt
- ✓ 2 TBSP garlic oil
- ✓ 1 cup mozzarella cheese
- ✓ 1 cup low carbohydrate tomato sauce

1) Preheat oven to 375 degrees. Pound/tenderize chicken breasts.

2) In a container, mix together parmesan cheese, Italian seasoning, and pork rinds. Add chicken breasts and shake until covered.

3) Place coated chicken on a roaster rack on top of a baking sheet. Sprinkle approximately ½ cup mozzarella cheese on top of each chicken breast.

4) Cook for 30-45 minutes or until the chicken measures 160 degrees on the meat thermometer.

5) Take zucchinis and shave into noodles with a peeler. Add garlic salt and oil to zoodles and toss. Set aside.

6) Remove chicken from oven and serve with zoodles.

3) Italian Parmesan Pork Cutlets

Ingredients
- ✓ *6 pork cutlets*
- ✓ *1/2 cup parmesan cheese*
- ✓ *1/2 cup Italian dressing*
- ✓ *Favorite seasonings*

1) Heat frying pan over medium heat.
2) Pour Italian dressing into one bowl and add parmesan cheese into a separate bowl.
3) Dip each cutlet into Italian dressing first and then into the parmesan cheese.
4) Cook in pan for approximately 15 minutes or until cooked through.

4) 5 Minute Cheese Fried Pizza

Ingredients
- ✓ 1 TBSP garlic olive oil
- ✓ 1/2 cup asiago cheese & 1 cup mozzarella cheese (or just 1 1/2 cup mozzarella)
- ✓ 1/3 cup tomato sauce
- ✓ Pizza/Italian seasoning
- ✓ Grated parmesan cheese

1) Heat pan over medium heat and add garlic olive oil. When pan is shiny, add mozzarella.

2) Use spatula to spread cheese evenly and cook for approximately three to five minutes while it melts and becomes dark around edges.

3) Once cheese has melted and started to brown, add tomato sauce and spread lightly with spoon.

4) Cook for approximately 1 minute.

5) Get the pizza unstuck from the pan without lifting it off completely.

6) Once pizza is free, you can tip the pan and slide it on a foil lined pan.

7) Sprinkle grated cheese and your preferred seasonings and allow to cool for about 1 minute.

5) Fried Cheddar Mexican Pizza

Ingredients

Taco Meat
- ½ pound ground beef
- 1/2 tsp paprika
- 1/2 tsp ground cumin
- 1 tsp chili powder
- 1/4 tsp garlic powder
- 1/2 tsp black pepper, ground
- 1/2 tsp pink Himalayan sea salt

Pizza
- 3/4 cup shredded cheddar cheese
- 1/2 cup four cheese Mexican blend

Toppings (this is all your choice!)
- Shredded lettuce
- Salsa
- Sour cream
- Picante/hot sauce
- Pico de gallo
- Shredded cheddar cheese
- Guacamole

1) For taco meat, brown ground beef in a skillet over medium high. Add 1/4 cup water and dry taco meat ingredients. Simmer for approximately 5 minutes and set aside.

2) For pizza, heat skillet over medium heat and add 2 TBSP olive oil. Quickly add Mexican blend to pan then cheddar on top once the pan is hot.

3) Shape edges of pizza into a circle using a spatula. Cook for about 4-5 minutes until easily lifted with a spatula. Use spatula to lift around all the edges until crust easily slides out. Slide onto plate and allow to cool.

4) Top pizza as desired and enjoy!

6) Nacho Chicken Casserole

Ingredients
- ✓ *1 3/4 pound boneless, skinless chicken thighs*
- ✓ *2 TBSP olive oil*
- ✓ *1 1/2 tsp chili seasoning*
- ✓ *1 cup tomatoes and green chilies*
- ✓ *4 ounces cream cheese*
- ✓ *1/4 cup sour cream*
- ✓ *4 ounces cheddar cheese*
- ✓ *1 medium-sized jalapeno pepper*
- ✓ *3 TBSP parmesan cheese*
- ✓ *16 ounces cauliflower*
- ✓ *Salt/pepper to taste*

1) Preheat oven to 375 degrees. Chop chicken into bite-sized chunks and season with chili seasoning, salt, and pepper.

2) Cook chicken over medium-high heat until brown on all sides.

3) Add sour cream, 3/4 of cheddar cheese, and cream cheese and stir until melted and mixed. Add tomatoes and green chilies and mix well.

4) Transfer chicken mixture from pan to casserole dish.

5) Steam cauliflower in microwave and use immersion blender to blend the cauliflower with cheese until it reaches mashed potato consistency. Season as desired with salt and pepper.

6) Cut jalapeno into chunks. Spread cauliflower mixture over top of chicken mixture and sprinkle jalapeno on top. Bake for 15-20 minutes or until it starts to brown on top and the jalapenos are cooked.

7) Keto-Style Kung Pao Chicken

Ingredients
Chicken
- 1/4 cup peanuts
- 2 large spring onions
- 2 medium chicken thighs, skin on, bone in
- 1/2 medium green pepper
- 1 tsp ground ginger
- 4 red chilies, de-seeded
- Salt/pepper to taste

Sauce
- 2 tsp rice wine vinegar
- 1 TBSP reduced sugar ketchup
- 1 TBSP soy sauce
- 2 TBSP chili garlic paste
- 10 drops liquid stevia
- 1/2 tsp maple extract
- 2 tsp sesame oil

1) Debone chicken and cut into bite-sized pieces. Season with ground ginger, salt, and pepper.

2) Heat pan over medium-high heat and once hot, add chicken. Allow chicken to cook until browned.

3) Chop and prepare veggies and chilies and set aside.

4) Combine all sauce ingredients together and mix well.

5) Once chicken is browned, stir everything together and allow to cook for a few more minutes. Add veggies and peanuts and allow to cook down for approximately 3-4 minutes.

6) Add sauce and allow to boil down slightly- should be slightly sticky when done.

8) Curry-Coconut Chicken Tenders
Ingredients
Chicken
- 5 deboned, skin-on chicken thighs
- 1/2 cup crumbled pork rinds
- 1 large egg
- 1/2 tsp coriander
- 2 tsp curry powder
- 1/4 tsp each garlic powder and onion powder
- 1/2 cup shredded, unsweetened coconut
- Salt/Pepper to taste

Sauce
- 1/4 cup each mayo and sour cream
- 1 1/2 tsp mango extract
- 2 TBSP sugar-free ketchup
- 1/2 tsp each garlic powder, ground ginger, and red pepper flakes
- 1/4 tsp cayenne pepper
- 7 drops liquid stevia

1) Preheat oven to 400 degrees and prepare a cookie sheet and wire rack. In a shallow bowl, beat the egg.

2) In large resealable bag, place shredded coconut, spices, and pork rinds.

3) Debone chicken thighs, taking care to leave skin on. Cut into strips- you should average around four strips per thigh.

4) Dip strips, a few at a time, in the egg and then place in bag and toss. Place on wire rack over cookie sheet.

5) Place cookie sheet with wire rack in oven for approximately 15 minutes. Remove and flip each strip and bake for another 20 minutes.

6) While your chicken is cooking, make the sauce by mixing together all of the listed ingredients and set aside until chicken is ready.

7) When chicken is done, remove from oven and serve. Enjoy!

9) Asian Grilled Keto-Style Short Ribs

Ingredients

Ribs/Marinade
- 1/4 cup soy sauce
- 2 TBSP fish sauce
- 2 TBSP rice vinegar
- 6 large short ribs

Asian Spice Rub
- 1/2 tsp each minced garlic, onion powder, sesame seed, and red pepper flakes
- 1/4 tsp cardamom
- 1 tsp ground ginger
- 1 TBSP salt

1) Mix together rice vinegar, fish sauce, and soy sauce. If desired, add sesame and olive oil to marinade.
2) Lay short ribs in a casserole dish and pour over marinade- allow to sit for 45 to 60 minutes.
3) Mix together spice rub.
4) Empty marinade from casserole dish and pour spice mixture evenly over both sides of ribs.
5) Heat grill and grill about 3-5 minutes per side depending upon thickness. Serve and enjoy!

10) Bacon Cheeseburger Stuffed with Cheese

Ingredients
- 8 ounces ground beef
- 2 precooked slices bacon
- 2 ounce cheddar cheese
- 1 ounce mozzarella cheese
- 1 tsp each salt and Cajun seasoning
- ½ tsp pepper
- 1 TBSP butter

1) Mix all spices together with the ground beef to season.
2) Prepare cheeses by cubing 1 ounce mozzarella and slicing 2 ounces of cheddar.
3) Form patties with ground beef, placing mozzarella cubes inside, closing beef around cheese.
4) Heat 1 TBSP butter in pan (per patty) and wait until hot and bubbly. Add patty to pan.
5) Cover and allow to cook for 2-3 minutes.
6) Flip burger and place cheddar on top. Cover again and let cook for approximately 1-2 minutes longer or until desired temp is reached.
7) Chop bacon in half and place on top of patty.

11) Reverse Seared Ribeye
Ingredients
- *3 TBSP bacon fat*
- *2 medium ribeye steaks*
- *Salt/pepper to taste*

1) Preheat oven to 250 degrees. Place steaks on wire rack on top of cookie sheet. Season with salt and pepper to taste.

2) Bake in oven until an internal temp of 123 degrees is reached- approximately 40-45 minutes.

3) Allow steaks to rest for only a few minutes.

4) Heat bacon grease in cast iron skillet and wait until extremely hot. Place steaks in skillet and sear for 30-45 seconds on each side.

5) Allow to rest for 2-3 minutes and serve.

12) Blackberry Chipotle Chicken Wings

Ingredients
- ✓ *20 chicken wings*
- ✓ *1/2 cup blackberry chipotle jam*
- ✓ *1/2 cup water*
- ✓ *Salt/pepper to taste*

1) Place chicken wings on cutting board, and detach the drumette from the wing.

2) Once you have detached the drumette from the wing, locate the secondary "V" between the wing and the tip. Cut off the wing tip and freeze to make broth later on.

3) Combine 1/2 cup blackberry chipotle jam, 1/2 cup water and whisk to combine. Add 2/3 marinade with chicken wings and salt/pepper in container and allow to sit for at least 30 minutes.

4) Preheat oven to 400 degrees. Once chicken is finished marinating, lay on a wire rack over a cookie sheet. Bake for 15 minutes then flip and increase oven temp to 425 degrees. Brush remainder of marinade over wings and bake for 20-30 minutes or until crispy.

13) Sage and Orange Duck Breast

Ingredients
- ✓ *2 TBSP butter*
- ✓ *1 TBSP sweetener*
- ✓ *16 ounce duck breast*
- ✓ *1 TBSP heavy cream*
- ✓ *1/2 tsp orange extract*
- ✓ *1 cup spinach*
- ✓ *1/4 tsp sage*

1) Score skin on top of duck breast and season on both sides with salt/pepper.

2) Place pan over medium-low heat, adding butter and sweetener. Allow to cook down until butter is slightly brown. Once butter is dark and golden, add orange extract and sage. Allow to cook until butter has reached a deep amber color.

3) Get out a cold pan and place duck breast in it. Set pan over medium-high heat on the stove. After 3-5 minutes, flip duck breast.

4) Add heavy cream to the butter mixture and stir well. Pour over duck breast and allow to mix with duck fat. Cook 3-5 more minutes.

5) Wilt spinach in the pan used to make sauce.

6) Allow duck to rest for 2-3 minutes and then slice and place on top of wilted spinach with sauce. Enjoy!

14) Italian Stuffed Meatballs

Ingredients

- ✓ 1 1/2 pound 80/20 ground beef
- ✓ 1/2 tsp Italian seasoning
- ✓ 2 large eggs
- ✓ 1 tsp oregano
- ✓ 2 tsp minced garlic
- ✓ 1/2 tsp onion powder
- ✓ 1/2 cup sliced olives
- ✓ 3 TBSP flaxseed meal
- ✓ 3 TBSP tomato paste
- ✓ 1/2 cup mozzarella cheese
- ✓ 1 tsp Worcestershire sauce
- ✓ Salt/pepper to taste

1) In large bowl, add ground beef, garlic and onion powder, Italian seasoning, and oregano. Mix well.

2) Add eggs, flaxseed meal, Worcestershire sauce and tomato paste to meat and mix well.

3) Slice olives into small pieces and add to meat mixture. Add mozzarella cheese to mixture and mix well.

4) Preheat oven to 400 degrees and then start forming the meatballs. You should have approximately 20 total. Lay on a cookie sheet covered with foil.

5) Bake for 16-20 minutes or until done to your liking.

15) Bacon Cheeseburger Soup

Ingredients

Nuggets

- ✓ 24 ounces cut chicken thighs
- ✓ 1 1/2 ounce pork rinds
- ✓ 1 large egg
- ✓ 1/4 cup each almond and flaxseed meals
- ✓ Zest from one lime
- ✓ 1/4 tsp each of salt, pepper, paprika, and chili powder
- ✓ 1/8 tsp each of garlic powder, onion powder, and cayenne powder

Sauce

- ✓ 1/2 cup mayo
- ✓ 1/2 tsp red chili flakes
- ✓ 1/8 tsp cumin
- ✓ 1/4 tsp garlic powder

- ✓ 1 TBSP lime juice

- ✓ 1/2 medium avocado

1) Preheat oven to 400 degrees. Dry chicken with paper towels, cut into chunks, and set aside.

2) In food processor, combine almond meal, lime zest, spices, flax meal, and pork rinds. Pulse until you have fine crumbs.

3) Put crumbs in one bowl. In a second bowl, crack one egg and scramble completely.

4) Dip chicken in egg mixture and then dip into crumb mixture making sure to coat both sides evenly. Lay on foil lined cookie sheet. (Tip: If you need more egg wash, add 1-2 teaspoons of water to the scrambled egg).

5) Bake for 15-18 minutes or until nuggets are golden brown and meat is cooked.

   While nuggets cool, put together the sauce ingredients and mix well. Enjoy!

Chapter 11

Convenient Keto Snacks

When you think about snacking and a ketogenic diet, they don't really seem to go together, do they? However, believe it or not, there are plenty of low carbohydrate snacks available. Whether you want something you can grab and go or something you can throw together in the kitchen on a Saturday afternoon, you'll find many great options below:

1) Vegetables and dip: this is a great snack that you can eat at home or grab and go. Some of my favorite veggies include broccoli, green and/or red peppers, and cucumbers. My favorite "go-to" dressing is ranch. I try to stay away from the so-called "low-fat" ones because they are typically high in carbohydrates. I always keep some smaller, travel containers so that I can take my snacks with me.

2) Pepperoni Slices: this is another one of my favorite snacks either alone or paired with cheese. However, I do have to watch my calories with this one because they really can add up quick.

3) Cheese and Deli meat wraps: Similar to the pepperoni slices, these are super quick and super easy to make when I'm looking for a low carbohydrate snack. I just take some cheese and wrap it up, using a toothpick, with some of my favorite deli meats such as roast beef, turkey, or ham.

4) Peanuts: of course, these probably aren't exactly one of the best ketogenic snacks, but they're okay in moderation. A ¼ cup of peanuts have around 3 grams of net carbohydrates.

5) Almonds: Almonds are another great snack choice because they only have 2.5 grams of net carbs for ¼ cup.

6) Hard-boiled eggs: these are portable, quick, and easy- and they are also incredibly healthy. I try to always keep a few hard-boiled eggs in my refrigerator so that I have them on hand when I want a quick, low carbohydrate snack.

7) Small salad: these are always a great option for a ketogenic snack, whether you want some mixed greens with olive oil or something a little more complex like a chef's salad.

8) String Cheese: this is a super simple snack all on it's own or paired with some deli meat or pepperoni slices. However, make sure that you choose the full-fat versions. The low fat options usually mean higher carbs and unhealthy fillers.

9) Pork Rinds: There are lots of options to choose from. Though it may sound weird to buy microwavable pork rinds, believe it or not, they are actually quite delicious. Plus, you can make some really great pork rind nachos or even crumble them up and make some breadcrumbs for fried chicken.

10) Celery and PB or Cream Cheese: Celery is very low in calories. Add a topping such as cream cheese or even peanut butter and you have a yummy and filling snack.

There are many more options for keto snacks out there, these are just some of my favorites. I encourage you to do some experimenting on your own and see what you can come up with!

Part Three

Sticking with the Ketogenic Diet

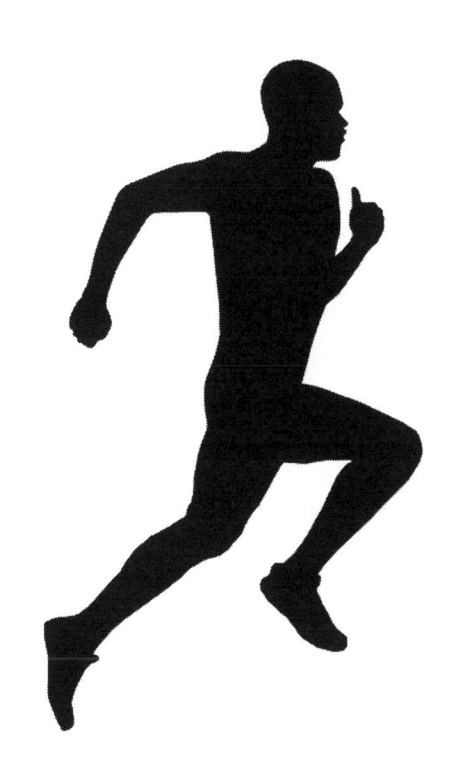

Chapter 12
Goals & Mindset for Maintaining a Ketogenic Diet

A low carbohydrate, or ketogenic, diet is an excellent way to achieve rapid results with weight loss while at the same time feeling healthier, eliminating your unhealthy cravings, and still being able to eat the foods that you enjoy. Still, as with any other diet, restrictions can sometimes be a source of frustration and there will be times when you may struggle. In this chapter, you will find some tips to keep you motivated to maintain your ketogenic diet.

1) Reach out for support.

Things are so much easier to do when you have the support of those who are doing the same thing. If you have friends that also want to lose weight and get healthy, encourage them to join you on your ketogenic quest. Together you'll both be able to experience the highs and the lows and will be able to swap recipes.

You can also look online for support. There are so many people who are currently using the ketogenic diet and sharing their experiences with the world. There are many great ketogenic diet forums online that can provide inspiration and answers to any questions you might have.

2) Accentuate the positive.

When you find yourself longing for a piece of cake or a cold beer, instead redirect your focus on what you've already achieved. Don't just think about the weight that you've lost, but your overall health. Chances are you are already feeling much more energetic than ever before. You're also probably sleeping much better. Consider how you're feeling now versus how you felt before you started on the ketogenic lifestyle. You're on your way to a better body and life.

3) Deal with setbacks right away.

Everyone falls off the wagon once in a while and eats or drinks something they are not supposed to - especially when just getting started. Don't beat yourself up about it and walk away. The ketogenic diet is more than a diet, it's a lifestyle.

Yes, when you overload on the carbs, your body will be thrown out of ketosis and you'll need a few days to get back into it. It's really easy to get back on track, but you must do it as soon as possible so that your body isn't completely out of whack. Just make sure you are not cheating on a regular basis.

Chapter 13
A System for Easily Preparing Your Meals for the Week

Ketogenic diet meal preparation doesn't have to be complicated. If you can take a little extra time on the weekends, you can easily prepare all of your meals for the week.

4) Cook all meat on Sunday and eat with veggies during the week. You can prepare veggies fresh when you're ready to eat or you can make them ahead of time.

5) Prepare a batch of cauli-rice each week to keep on hand. Having it ready ahead of time is extremely convenient. Plus, cauli-rice is an all-around good thing because it can be used as a side or even as a quick grab and go breakfast.

6) Chop fresh veggies ahead of time. Cut them up and place them in mason jars or other types of containers to create some simple grab and go salads. Top them with protein and fat when ready to eat.

7) Pre-cook and freeze veggies. Visit your local farmer's market and purchase fresh veggies when they are in season. Blanch them until half done, but still crisp. In most cases 1-3 minutes is enough time. Rinse well and drain before freezing in single portion bags. When you prepare your veggies this way, they take very little time to cook when you're ready to eat.

8) Cook your meat in a pressure or slow cooker. This will result in large amounts of meat at one time that you can use during the week for various meals. Plus, you can freeze any excess for

later use. I love making a big pork or turkey roast at the beginning of the week.

9) Save bone broths and use for a flavor boost. Bone broth is a great way to add flavor to your dishes without having to use extra herbs and spices. I often cook my veggies in bone broth to make them taste great.

10) Make some homemade pesto sauce and keep it in the fridge. It only takes a few minutes to prepare and will add lots of flavor to your dishes.

11) When you are heading out, take a lunch box with you. This will limit temptations and ensure that you always have keto-friendly foods with you.

12) Keep keto-friendly ingredients on hand that you can make quick meals out of such as cream, butter, avocados, meats, eggs, cheeses, and non-starchy veggies.

13) Make some keto-friendly snacks ahead of time and put them in the fridge or your car. These can include: hard boiled eggs, avocados, homemade keto bars, nuts and nut butters, and even fat bombs.

Chapter 14
How to Deal with Temptations & Sugar Cravings

Sugar addiction is a real issue. The effects that refined sugar have on your body are very similar to those that serious drugs do. Once you are addicted to sugar, you are now locked into that cycle of sugar highs followed by slumps/cravings for more. At some point your health will begin to deteriorate.

The best way to break this cycle is to cut refined sugar from your diet. While ketogenic/low carbohydrate diets are one of the best ways to do this, you should be aware that the change is not going to be instantaneous. You're going to experience some pretty significant sugar cravings. At some point, your body will adapt to the low carbohydrate and sugar-free lifestyle and you will no longer experience these strong cravings.

In the meantime, you're going to need some help for battling those cravings until your body has reached full ketosis. Following are 15 tips for getting through this time.

1) Make sure to eat protein with every meal.

When you haven't had enough protein, you will often begin to feel sugar cravings. A decent amount of protein will keep you fuller much longer and will keep you from feeling that desire to consume sugary snacks. Additionally, the protein will keep your muscle mass from deteriorating when you are in ketosis.

2) Never be afraid of fats.

Even if you're following a different low-carbohydrate diet plan, you should never consume less than the recommended levels of fat. Typically, you should consume no less than 50 grams of fat per day. Eating something with a high fat content can help to alleviate any sugar cravings.

3) Never starve yourself.

One of the best things about deciding to go on a ketogenic diet is that you will naturally begin to feel less hungry, therefore, eating less. However, never purposefully skip meals or reduce calories in addition to eating low carbohydrate meals. This can cause you to have strong sugar cravings and result in you falling off of your diet completely.

4) Eat more often.

When you're on a ketogenic diet and you find yourself frequently craving sugar, rearrange your eating schedule. Instead of eating three meals, have six small meals every day. You could also try eating a low carbohydrate snack in between meals. Eating more often will keep your body fueled and you will be less likely to develop cravings.

5) Make sure to choose whole foods instead of processed ones.

Always choose whole foods over processed foods. Processed foods are often full of empty calories and chemicals. Whole foods are much more nutritious and often contain more fiber, making you feel fuller for much longer.

6) Always drink plenty of water.

When your body is burning fat for fuel, the amount of water your body needs is increased, so make sure you are staying hydrated. I aim for a gallon of water every day. Drinking more water will also make you feel more alert and less tired throughout the day.

7) Take supplements to counteract your sugar cravings.

There are some specific supplements that can help you to counteract sugar cravings. These include: omega 3, green tea extract, L-Carnitine, chromium, and L-Glutamine. **You can find these supplements here http://amzn.to/1KfzSWS**

8) Always approach the artificial sweeteners cautiously.

The name says it all: artificial sweeteners are artificial. Though they do not have an immediate effect on the glucose levels in your blood, they are still not great. Many people say that artificial sweeteners cause their body to want the real thing. So, if this is the case for you, it's best to stay off of them. Then again, others say that just a little sweetener counteracts their sugar cravings. So, this is entirely your call. You will have to experiment and see which works best for you.

9) Reduce or eliminate caffeine.

Caffeine has an effect on your blood sugar levels and can result in strong sugar cravings. So, if you're someone that must have your coffee and you're always struggling with craving sugar, try to reduce or even eliminate your caffeine consumption and see if it helps. Try replacing your morning coffee with some Yerba Mate tea instead to slowly begin reducing your caffeine consumption.

10)   Make sure to get plenty of sleep.

Not getting a sufficient amount of sleep may cause your body to demand a quick fix for the lack of energy in the form of sugar. Therefore, if you regularly miss out on sleep, you're likely to find it difficult to stay on track with your ketogenic diet. Come up with a sleep schedule and try to stick to it regularly, even on the weekends.

11)   Avoid temptations whenever possible.

We all know that sugary foods are very tempting. The cake displays or the candy aisle in the grocery store can easily grab you and get you off track. Try avoiding those situations and the places that can cause you to be tempted. Make sure that you do not keep sugary foods in your home. After all, it takes much more willpower to control your cravings when it is easily accessible. I love shopping for ketogenic foods on Amazon.com because I am not forced to walk by tempting foods in the grocery store.

12)   Get enough exercise.

This one may seem pretty obvious. Everyone should be exercising, right? However, this one is included here because exercise raises the serotonin levels in your brain. You already know that sugar does the same thing. So, by exercising, you're filling that void. You should participate in intensive exercise such as high intensity interval training, or HIIT, or even heavy weight-lifting in order to effectively and quickly raise your serotonin levels. When I experience sugar cravings, I jump rope for 5-10 minutes and this is usually just enough to limit the craving.

13) Never reward yourself with food - you're not a dog.

Early in life, we learn that sweet foods are "treats." Though it can be quite difficult to break away from this thought process, you must find something else instead. Choose a different, non-sugary food that you enjoy - or an activity that you enjoy doing instead of eating. Another option is to treat yourself to a small shopping spree. I will sometimes buy a new book, makeup, or electronic gadgets to reward myself for sticking to my ketogenic diet.

14) Avoid giving in to emotional hunger.

Many people have emotional triggers that result in consumption of sugar. Maybe it's anxiety, shame, anger, or even stress. Find out what your triggers are and try to get to the underlying causes of those triggers so you can find more constructive ways of dealing with them. If your emotional issues are severe, you may need to address them with a professional or even utilize some self-help resources.

15) Follow the ketogenic guidelines to the letter.

All diets can work, but only if you're willing to work with them. When you decide to go on a ketogenic diet, you must make sure that you're following the guidelines exactly and that you are fully committed. These diet plans have been carefully constructed, so try not to stray from them.

Chapter 15
How to Handle Social Pressure

Chances are there are going to be some people in your life who are going to pick fun at you when you tell them you have decided to go on a ketogenic diet.

When I was first told about the ketogenic diet, I had the same exact thought that most people do: meat and cheese all the time- yuck! However, I took a step back and did some research. In fact, I spent lots of time researching, reading studies, academic papers, and so much more.

Now, after all that research, I am a believer in the ketogenic diet as a way of life. I found out that it's so much more than just meats and cheeses - veggies are encouraged too! So, I decided to jump on board with this diet and I feel better than I ever have before.

Of course, when you're doing something new that makes you feel good, there are going to be some people in your life that try to rain on your parade. Here are eight of the most common pressures that I've seen and how you can respond to them.

1) Low carbohydrate diets are horrible for you!

While some low carbohydrate diets are unhealthy, not all of them are created equally. The term ketogenic is a scientific one and describes a way of eating that eliminates carbohydrates. On a ketogenic diet, your body is running off ketones and fats, not carbs. Therefore, ingesting carbs is not necessary. Ingesting low amounts of carbs when your body is using carbs and glucose for energy is when you can run into trouble and why people say that low carbohydrate diets are bad.

2) Your body needs carbohydrates for energy!

Even on a low carbohydrate diet, you're still getting carbohydrates in the form of veggies. However, our bodies were not built to run on carbohydrates and the truth is, you're not depriving your body of energy at all by eliminating carbohydrates. Our bodies prefer to run on their own fuel from fats, known as ketones. This is the reason why those who have reduced or even eliminated carbohydrates are able to concentrate and think much clearer. For the areas of your brain requiring glucose, your body will turn the protein you consume, into glucose through gluconeogenesis. Your body does not need a lot of carbohydrates to run, even if you are extremely active.

3) There are so many better ways for you to lose weight!

Sure, there are many ways to lose weight, but the ketogenic diet provides much more than just weight loss. Those who are on ketogenic diets are not necessarily doing it just to lose a few pounds. Sure, it's a great bonus and a way that you can measure your progress, but many do it for the health benefits. Physicians are prescribing the ketogenic diet to cancer patients, Alzheimer's patients, and those who have MS and other conditions. It has been extremely effective at treating these conditions. Business owners and employees also use the ketogenic diet to have more energy, focus, and mental clarity.

4) Do you just eat bacon all day long?

I very rarely eat bacon. This is one of the worst generalizations of all. Those who are on a ketogenic diet eat more whole foods such as veggies. In fact, keto people probably eat more veggies than most! We also can eat berries. The things we don't eat are sugary fruits and starchy veggies. We're not giving them up because we have to - but because we don't want them anymore.

5) It's not healthy to be eating 5000 calories a day - how can you possibly lose any weight?

Ketogenic diets are naturally low in calories. This is another very irritating generalization that low carbohydrate diets get. People assume that keto dieters are consuming tons of calories. However, the reality is that it is hard to eat tons of calories when you eliminate carbohydrates because most of the calories that people are consuming come from the carbs. Personally, I have an extremely hard time consuming 1500 calories a day and often have to push myself.

6) Sugar alcohols are just as bad as fake sugar, right?

I'm not really sure, but most keto people are not consuming sugar alcohols. Sure, there are lots of popular diets that include fake sweeteners and fake ingredients. However, for most of us following a ketogenic diet, we are shopping in the produce, dairy, and meat sections of the store. Since milk is high in sugar, almond milk is a great alternative. Also, eggs and cheeses are highly encouraged. I very rarely go down the aisles of the store - which means no fake foods.

7) Consuming so much fat is horrible for you and will kill you.

The truth is, fat does not cause a person to be fat. The ingredients in a ketogenic diet are actually "good fats" and are healthy for you. People on ketogenic diets often choose real butter over fake margarine. We like to cook in coconut oil. We choose grass fed meats because of the omega-3s and good fats. We choose uncured, nitrate-free bacon and deli meats because the nitrates and other junk in processed meats are not healthy.

8) You've got to be starving all the time!

Nope, not at all. The truth is, when you're on a ketogenic diet, you're rarely hungry. Carbohydrates cause you to feel hungry all the time and therefore, you eat more. Without the carbohydrates, I'm actually eating much less and I don't feel the need to snack all the time. My cravings have disappeared and I'm eating whole foods and watching my weight effortlessly shed away.

The truth of the matter is this: a basic ketogenic diet will include plenty of veggies, meats, nuts, and some dairy and fruit. There is no processed stuff, sugars, or grains when eating a ketogenic diet. We consume 20 to 60 grams of net carbohydrates daily - that's carbs minus fiber - and once you have eliminated grains, this is pretty easy to do.

People often tell you that you shouldn't "diet," but simply make good choices. That's what the ketogenic diet is all about. Keto people are eating good, real foods. Eating ketogenic shouldn't even be called a diet, but a way of life.

So, next time someone tries to tell you that your diet is going to kill you, just tell them that you're much more worried about their diet than your own and they should at least consider learning more about the ketogenic diet.

Chapter 16
Options for Eating Out at Restaurants

These days, everyone is so busy and many people dine out quite often. Others might have careers that require them to dine out with clients. Either way, dining out can lead to carbohydrate overload. However, by simply using the same thought process that you use when eating at home, you can very easily find low carbohydrate options on any menu. Following are a few tips to help you stay true to your ketogenic diet when dining out.

1) Chinese Restaurants

Of course you know that Chinese food can be chock full of fresh ingredients and wonderful veggies. However, the noodles and the rice in these dishes cause the carbohydrate content to skyrocket. By skipping the noodles, rice, wontons, fried noodles, breaded items, and most of the sauces, you can pretty much stay on track. Still, you must consider any hidden carbohydrates when you're placing your order. While chicken and broccoli without rice sounds like an excellent keto choice, you must be aware that often the sauce will contain cornstarch.

Here's what you should order when eating at a Chinese restaurant:

- a) Soups: Hot and Sour, Chicken Broth with Scallions, and Egg Drop

- b) Egg Rolls: Open the eggroll and eat the inside- skip the wrap

- c) Steamed foods without the sauce: Have a side of chicken broth or egg drop soup on the side and use it for your sauce

- d) Stir-fry: Order these dishes without starch or sugar

e) Egg Foo Young: Order without gravy

f) Mu Shu: Order without wrappers

g) Mongolian BBQ: This is often available at Chinese Buffets - choose your own veggies and meats and ask for no sauce

2) Italian Restaurants

When you think about Italian food, chances are you start thinking about crusty white bread, lots of pasta, and pizza. However, Italians don't really load up on carbohydrates as we tend to think. In Rome, the pizza is made on paper-thin crust, very light tomato sauce, and little cheese. This is not at all like the greasy pizza we have in America. Here are a few tips to keep you on the keto track when dining at an Italian restaurant:

a) Antipasti: this term refers to "before the meal" and options often include a variety of keto-friendly meats, cheeses, olives, and marinated veggies.

b) Italian Soups: Simple Veggie Soup, Italian Egg Drop Soup, Chicken Broth with Spinach, and Italian Wedding Soup without Pasta

c) Salads: Italian salads mostly contain dark greens, crushed garlic, and olive oil. You can add tomatoes and cheese if you like, but avoid the croutons.

d) Seafood: This is usually a great option to remain keto. You can also choose veal and chicken entrees with sauce on the side.

e) Pizza: You don't have to completely give up pizza. Enjoy just the toppings such as peppers, broccoli, onions, spinach, and cheese. Leave your crust behind.

3) Mexican Restaurants

You probably already know that Mexican food consists of beans, tortillas, rice, corn, tamales, tacos, enchiladas, and burritos that are loaded with carbohydrates. So, what can you do? The trick is to make sure that you count your carbohydrates and consider what is inside the tortillas, tacos, and other dishes. Here are some tips on what to order when eating Mexican:

   a) Guacamole and cucumber chips: avocado is great for your heart, so eat as much as you like. You can use cucumber chips to dip or just eat it with a spoon.

   b) Ensalada: Salads are great choices for an appetizer. However, you should tell them to put it on a plate instead of in the tortilla shell.

   c) Grilled veggies and proteins: chicken dishes with grilled veggies, grilled seafood with just a light salsa, and Carne Asada, or grilled steak & Mexican spices are all excellent choices.

   d) Fajitas: Yes, even on a low carbohydrate diet, you can still enjoy fajitas- at least the insides - just skip the tortillas.

   e) Machaca: this is a common Mexican breakfast comprised of beef, veggies, and eggs and is a low carbohydrate dream.

Fast Food Restaurants

When it comes to eating at fast food restaurants, most people are lost when it comes to choosing low carbohydrate options. However, it is possible to stay true to your keto diet when grabbing a quick bite to eat. Here are a few tips to help you out:

a) Grilled Chicken: this makes a great meal, along with lettuce, tomato, and cheese.

b) Grilled Burgers: ask them to leave it off the bun and top it with plenty of pickles, onions, lettuce, and tomato.

c) Salads: This is always a great option. Add a protein such as cheese and eggs, chicken, or even steak. Choose a vinaigrette or low fat dressing.

d) Get rid of the shell: just as the inside of burgers works well for a meal, the inside of tacos works well too - just don't eat the shell.

e) Breakfast muffin without the muffin: Order your breakfast sandwiches without the bread - or just throw it away when you open it. The restaurants in my local area will often wrap it in a piece of lettuce if you request no bread.

f) Sub sandwiches: make your sub sandwich into a salad by eating the insides and skipping the roll.

Though staying true to your keto diet when eating out seems like a daunting task, as you can see, it is very possible. You just have to be aware of the carbohydrate content of foods and make sure that you do what you can to avoid those carbs whenever possible. With these tips, you can easily find something to eat on any menu.

Conclusion/Challenge

Congratulations for reaching this point!

You have come further than most people. You should now know all about how the ketogenic diet works, how to get started, and how to stick with it.

However, it is not enough to just know the information. Now it is all on you to get started with the ketogenic diet and to achieve your goals.

I have a challenge for you.

For the next 30 days, I want you to stick to eating a ketogenic diet. If you don't like it after those 30 days, you can quit and go back to eating your normal diet. However, I can guarantee that you will feel so, SO much better. You probably won't ever want to go back to your old eating ways.

Sure, the comments from people can be annoying at times and that is something that you will have to get used to. But if you can stick to the diet for 30 days, I can almost guarantee you will lose weight quickly as long as you are not over-consuming calories. And guess what? You probably won't even feel like you're dieting because you will be eating foods that satiate your hunger and cravings. It's a win-win.

So right after reading this, I want you to go out and buy some fresh ketogenic foods and supplements to make this process as easy as possible. You will also need to figure out your target caloric intake and come up with a meal plan that will be easy to stick to.

If you'd like to order anything from Amazon, I would highly recommend the items on my Amazon store @ http://amzn.to/1KfzSWS I have been using them for years and have had great results!

Half the battle is having the right foods around you so you are not tempted to stray from the diet. Fill your house, car, and workplace with keto-friendly foods and snacks and you are virtually guaranteed to stick to the challenge.

Thanks again for reading and goodluck on your ketogenic journey!

Want 4 Free Reports That Will Make The Ketogenic Diet a Breeze?

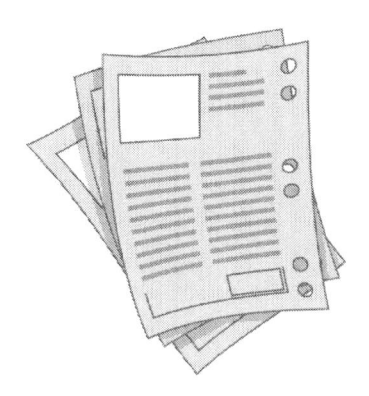

$17 Value!

The #1 reason people don't stick to a ketogenic diet is because they are tired of eating the same things over and over. That is why I have prepared 4 FREE PDF reports that will make sure you never get tired of sticking to the ketogenic diet.

I have taken the grocery list and recipes found in this book and have compiled them all into printable files that you can download, print, and take with you to the grocery store or kitchen to ensure that you always have variety and tasty foods in your diet.

Go to **http://bit.ly/1V24Kjf** to instantly download your $17 gift

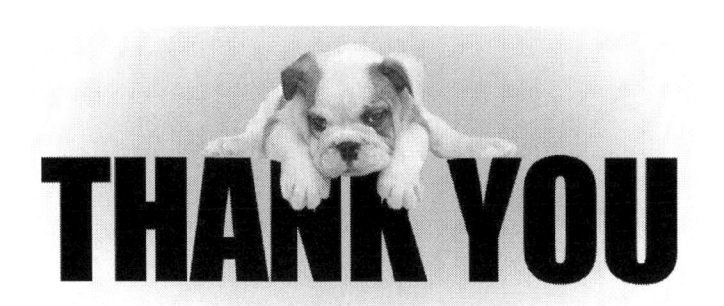

Thank You For Downloading My Book!

I really appreciate all of your feedback and I love hearing what you have to say.

I need your input to make the next version better.

Please leave me a helpful review on Amazon letting me know what you thought of the book.

Thanks so much!!!
- Maria Lively

Made in the USA
San Bernardino, CA
29 September 2016